Complete Guide
ACUPUNCTURE AND REFLEXOLOGY

Journey To Unlocking Holistic Healing & Wellness, Navigate Key Points, Target Ailments, Focus On Total Well-Being And Techniques For A Balanced Life

DR. POWELL SHIELDS

Copyright © 2023, Dr. Powell Shields

All rights reserved. Except for brief quotations incorporated in critical reviews and certain other noncommercial uses permitted by copyright law, without the publisher's prior written consent, no portion of this publication may be reproduced, distributed, or transmitted in any form or by any means, including photocopying, recording, or other electronic or mechanical methods.

DISCLAIMER:

The content presented in this book is for general educational purposes only. The content should not be considered as a substitute for professional medical advice, diagnosis, or treatment.

The author is not affiliated with any individual, organization, website, product, or entity that might be mentioned in this book. Any references made are for informational purposes only and do not imply endorsement. The author does not endorse or recommend any specific tests, physicians, products, procedures, opinions, or other information that may be mentioned in this book.

Readers are advised to consult with their healthcare professionals for advice and guidance regarding their individual health concerns. This book is not intended as a self-reliance guide, and the author disclaims any responsibility for any adverse effects or consequences resulting from the use of information presented in this book.

Medical knowledge is constantly evolving, and new information may emerge that could change the accuracy or relevance of the information provided in this book. The author assumes no responsibility for errors or omissions and is not liable for any damages resulting from the use of information contained herein.

DETAILED FACTS ABOUT THIS BOOK

The "Complete Guide to Acupuncture and Reflexology" is a priceless tool for deciphering the subtleties of these age-old Chinese medical techniques. The book begins with an examination of the fundamental ideas of Traditional Chinese Medicine (TCM) and then dives into the important role that energy, or Qi, plays in acupuncture and reflexology, giving readers a thorough grasp of these practices' beginnings and development.

This book provides a thorough understanding of the fundamentals of acupuncture by explaining the theories underlying the age-old modality, the mapping of meridians and acupoints, and the instruments and methods used. Fundamentals of reflexology are covered concurrently, providing information on how to map reflex zones on the hands, feet, and ears as well as the methods and advantages of this complementary therapy.

This book explains the processes underlying the synergy between acupuncture and reflexology and looks at the illnesses that both therapies can effectively treat, including pain management, stress, anxiety, digestive disorders, and infertility. It highlights how these two approaches complement one another and highlights how they can work together to promote holistic recovery.

A major subject is the incorporation of reflexology and acupuncture into regular wellness routines, highlighting their significance for holistic health. Beyond the physical, this book explores the mind-body link using traditional disciplines like breath work and meditation in addition to other methods.

Through practical considerations, this guide offers readers a tangible grasp of the transformational power of acupuncture and reflexology by guiding them in selecting certified practitioners, navigating safety concerns, and presenting real-life case studies and success stories.

It also considers these techniques' future, looking at TCM trends, research developments, and their ongoing integration into contemporary healthcare.

The "Complete Guide to Acupuncture and Reflexology" is essentially a crucial handbook that bridges the gap between traditional knowledge and modern insight, making these profound therapeutic therapies useful and approachable in today's world.

TABLE OF CONTENTS

CHAPTER 1 10

OVERVIEW OF CHINESE TRADITIONAL MEDICINE 10

CHAPTER 2 14

BASICS OF ACUPUNCTURE 14

CHAPTER 3 20

FOUNDATIONS OF REFLEXOLOGY 20

CHAPTER 4 24

THE MECHANISMS OF ACUPUNCTURE AND REFLEXOLOGY 24

CHAPTER 5 28

ACUPUNCTURE-TREATED CONDITIONS 28

CHAPTER 6 34

CONDITIONS TREATED WITH REFLEXOLOGY 34

CHAPTER 7 38

INCLUDING REFLEXOLOGY AND ACUPUNCTURE IN WELLNESS PRACTICES 38

CHAPTER 8 .... **44**

SELECTING A PRACTITIONER AND SAFETY ISSUES **44**

CHAPTER 9 .... **48**

CASE STUDIES AND SUCCESS STORIES IN **48**

CHAPTER 10 .... **52**

ACUPUNCTURE AND REFLEXOLOGY'S FUTURE **52**

THE END **58**

CHAPTER 1

OVERVIEW OF CHINESE TRADITIONAL MEDICINE
Understanding The Fundamentals Of Traditional Chinese Medicine

Over thousands of years, Traditional Chinese Medicine (TCM) has developed into a complete and ancient medical system. TCM, which has its philosophical roots in Taoism, emphasizes the interconnection of all components by viewing the human body as a microcosm of the greater universe. Fundamentally, TCM is predicated on the harmony and balance of life energy within the body, to preserve homeostasis to attain the best possible health. This integrated method combines several techniques, including nutritional treatment, massage, herbal medicine, acupuncture, and forms of exercise like tai chi and qigong.

Understanding the body's life force, or Qi is one of the core ideas of TCM. TCM holds that Qi permeates the body's meridians, or passageways, controlling and sustaining the organs and tissues. The other fundamental idea of TCM philosophy is the harmony of Yin and Yang, the complimentary and opposing forces. It is thought that illness results from imbalances or disturbances in the flow of Qi, whereas health is a condition of dynamic equilibrium between these forces.

The Function of Qi (energy) in Reflexology and Acupuncture

Two main pillars of TCM, acupuncture, and reflexology, depend on Qi manipulation to reestablish equilibrium and enhance health. To stimulate or regulate the flow of Qi, acupuncture involves inserting tiny needles into predetermined sites throughout the body's meridians.

Acupuncture targets deficiencies or obstructions in the flow of energy, with each point representing a certain organ or system.

Conversely, reflexology maps particular spots on the hands, feet, and ears that correlate to various organs and systems throughout the body. Practitioners aim to promote the body's natural healing processes and improve Qi circulation by applying pressure or massage to these reflex sites.

The foundational idea of reflexology and acupuncture is that emotional or bodily suffering arises from Qi imbalances. Practitioners hope to ease symptoms, restore general health, and harmonize the flow of energy through these therapies.

A Synopsis of Acupuncture and Reflexology's Development

Acupuncture and reflexology originated in ancient China, where they were developed over many years. The origins of acupuncture may be traced to the Neolithic era, when its concepts and procedures were recorded in the Huangdi Neijing, also known as the Yellow Emperor's Inner Canon. A key component of TCM, acupuncture developed through time by absorbing fresh ideas and methods.

Although reflexology has its roots in ancient cultures, early Chinese, Indian, and Egyptian traditions are greatly influenced by the contemporary version. Pioneers such as William H. Fitzgerald and Eunice Ingham popularized the idea of reflexology zones on the feet in the early 1900s. Both reflexology and acupuncture are now widely accepted worldwide, and new research is proving their effectiveness and extending their uses outside of conventional contexts. The historical relevance of these age-old techniques is a monument to the timeless wisdom of Traditional Chinese Medicine, even as they continue to evolve.

CHAPTER 2

BASICS OF ACUPUNCTURE
The Principles Behind Acupuncture:

The ancient Chinese concept of harmonizing the body's vital force, or Qi (pronounced "chee"), is the foundation of acupuncture. Traditional Chinese medicine holds that illness or discomfort is caused by imbalances or disturbances in the Qi flow. By carefully placing tiny needles into particular locations along the body's meridians—which are thought of as energy pathways—acupuncture works to restore equilibrium. The foundation of the practice is the idea that many organs and functions are connected by these meridians, which permit the free passage of Qi to preserve health.

The concept of the body's Yin and Yang, which stand for opposing forces that, when in balance, promote general well-being, is also consistent with acupuncture. Acupuncturists base their treatment of a wide range of health issues on the core concepts of Qi manipulation and Yin and Yang balance.

Acupoints and Meridians: Mapping the Energy Routes in the Body

The pathways that Qi travels via inside the body are called meridians. These channels link different acupoints, or acupuncture points, where the placement of needles is done in a certain way to affect the flow of energy. Each meridian in the complex meridian system corresponds to a particular organ or physiological system. As an illustration, the lung meridian is connected to respiratory function, whereas the stomach meridian is linked to digesting.

Acupoints are chosen with great care according to the type of imbalance or illness. Acupuncturists select sites that will either stimulate or tonify Qi, fostering harmony and balance inside the body, using a thorough grasp of the meridian system. One of the most important aspects of the art and science of acupuncture is the accurate mapping of meridians and acupoints, which calls for a thorough comprehension of the fundamentals of traditional Chinese medicine.

Instruments and Methods Used in Acupuncture:

The tiny, sterile needle is the main instrument used in acupuncture. These needles come in a variety of lengths and thicknesses and are usually composed of stainless steel. Acupuncturists use several needling techniques, such as insertion, manipulation (such as mild twisting or twirling), and removal.

Achieving the intended therapeutic results depends critically on the depth and angle of the needle entry.

Aside from standard needling, alternative methods of acupuncture include moxibustion, which includes burning the herb mugwort next to acupoints to promote healing, and electroacupuncture, which involves applying a mild electrical current to the needles.

Acupuncturists may choose to include acupressure or cupping in their treatments. Every approach has a distinct function and is customized to meet the demands of the patient.

Acupuncture Safety and Hygiene Procedures:

In acupuncture therapy, maintaining hygienic conditions and safety is crucial. Acupuncturists follow stringent guidelines to stave against infections and foster hygienic conditions. Disposable, single-use needles are the norm to reduce the chance of infection. To maintain a sterile environment during treatments, practitioners also wear gloves and follow strict handwashing protocols.

To reduce the risk of infection, acupuncture clinics regularly sterilize all surfaces and equipment. In order to create a personalized treatment plan and ensure that acupuncture is a safe and suitable option, acupuncturists also inquire about a patient's past medical history, allergies, and general health.

Following safety and hygiene guidelines protects the health of people seeking this age-old type of treatment as well as the reputation of acupuncture practitioners.

CHAPTER 3

FOUNDATIONS OF REFLEXOLOGY
Overview of Reflexology

The holistic treatment technique known as reflexology is based on the theory that specific body parts—the hands, feet, and ears in particular—have reflex points that are associated with different organs and systems. Practitioners think they may promote balance and enhance energy flow within the relevant parts of the body by pressing on these exact places. The underlying tenet of reflexology is the idea that these zones represent the body and that by working with them, one can improve general health and well-being.

Mapping the Hand, Ear, and Foot Reflex Zones:

Understanding how the reflex zones on the hands, feet, and ears are distributed requires familiarity with reflexology charts. It is thought that particular organs, glands, and bodily parts correspond to each location. For example, the heel is connected to the lower back and bowels, the toes to the brain, and the ball of the foot to the heart and chest. The hands and ears also contain reaction zones that correspond to various body regions. Reflexologists need precise mapping to stimulate relevant reflex points to target specific health concerns and the appropriate locations.

Methods of Reflexology and Pressure Points:

Reflexology uses a range of ways to apply pressure to the reflex zones. Practitioners of thumb and finger techniques frequently use particular motions including rubbing, kneading, and circular motions. Reflexologists with experience can change the pressure they apply and modify their technique according to the demands and sensitivities of each client. Releasing tension, enhancing circulation, and invigorating the body's inherent healing mechanisms are the goals.

To achieve the intended therapeutic results, it is essential to comprehend the different types of pressure points and use the proper procedures.

The advantages of reflexology

Numerous possible advantages for both mental and physical health are linked to reflexology. Since the practice tries to promote relaxation and release tension in all parts of the body, stress reduction is one of its main benefits. Another typical result is improved circulation, which enhances the delivery of nutrients and oxygen to cells and organs. Regular reflexology sessions help many people find relief from specific diseases like headaches, intestinal problems, and chronic pain. Reflexology's supporters also assert that it helps balance hormones, raise energy levels, and improve the body's general sense of harmony.

In conclusion, reflexology uses reflex zones on the hands, feet, and ears to leverage the body's interconnection to provide a holistic approach to health and healing. Reflexologists seek to help people seeking a natural and non-invasive kind of therapy by promoting balance, relaxation, and well-being through precise mapping, skillful use of techniques, and knowledge of pressure points.

CHAPTER 4

THE MECHANISMS OF ACUPUNCTURE AND REFLEXOLOGY
Examining the Acupuncture Mechanisms:

An essential part of traditional Chinese medicine, acupuncture works by encouraging equilibrium and the unrestricted movement of life force, or "Qi," throughout the body. Thin needles are inserted into particular locations throughout the body's meridian channels in this age-old technique. These meridians are thought of as the pathways that Qi travels through.

Acupuncturists seek to balance out imbalances and bring the body back into harmony by applying pressure to particular meridians. Acupuncture uses carefully positioned needles to affect Qi flow, which is thought to control several physiological functions including immune system response, blood flow, and neurotransmitter release.

Acupuncture's effects go beyond the parameters of traditional Chinese medicine, according to science. According to research, acupuncture may alter the nervous system's function, altering neurotransmitters like dopamine and serotonin and producing endorphins, the body's natural analgesics. Furthermore, acupuncture might have anti-inflammatory properties, which would explain why it works so well for inflammatory disorders.

Recognizing the Effects of Reflexology on the Nervous System:

Another complementary therapy method is reflexology, which involves stimulating particular reflex spots on the hands, feet, and ears that represent various body organs and systems. The foundation of this holistic approach is the idea that these reflex locations are linked to different nerve terminals and energy channels.

Reflexologists work to enhance general health and encourage healing throughout the body by applying pressure or massage to these reflex sites.

The neurological system is significantly impacted by reflexology. Reflexology relieves tension and generates a relaxation response by stimulating the nerve terminals on the extremities. This could then have a beneficial effect on the autonomic nervous system, balancing the body's "fight or flight" reaction and encouraging rest and renewal. Furthermore, reflexology is said to improve blood circulation, which helps the body's natural healing processes and makes it easier for nutrients and oxygen to reach cells.

The Complementary Aspects Of Reflexology And Acupuncture

Although the methodologies and areas of concentration of reflexology and acupuncture vary, they are fundamentally similar in that they take a holistic approach to improving wellness.

Both approaches acknowledge how different body systems are interdependent and work to bring balance back for optimum performance.

Reflexology and acupuncture can work in tandem to treat a variety of medical conditions. Acupuncture's influence on the nervous system and its systemic effects on the body's energy flow can work in concert with reflexology's focused stimulation of particular reflex spots. When combined, they might improve the treatment's overall efficacy and offer a more all-encompassing strategy for health and well-being. By combining these techniques, people can receive a customized, all-encompassing approach to preserving equilibrium and taking care of certain health issues.

CHAPTER 5

ACUPUNCTURE-TREATED CONDITIONS
Acupuncture as a Pain Management Technique:

Pain management is one of the fields in which acupuncture is most widely used. Since ancient times, acupuncture has been used to treat a wide range of pains, from acute accidents to chronic illnesses like arthritis. Thin needles are inserted into predetermined bodily locations to trigger endorphin release and trigger the body's natural pain-relieving processes. In addition to treating the symptoms, this holistic approach seeks to address the underlying imbalances causing the discomfort. Many people use acupuncture as a supplemental or alternative pain management technique, reporting notable benefits in their general well-being and decreased dependency on prescription painkillers.

Acupuncture to Reduce Anxiety and Stress:

Stress and anxiety are common problems in today's world that have an impact on both physical and mental health.

Acupuncture promotes relaxation and balances the body's energy flow, providing a comprehensive approach to managing various disorders.

The goals of acupuncture practitioners are to balance the nervous system, lower cortisol levels, and improve general calm by focusing on particular acupuncture points associated with stress response and emotional well-being.

According to a plethora of research, acupuncture can be a beneficial part of an all-encompassing stress management strategy, giving people a safe, natural alternative to medication for reducing the negative effects of stress and anxiety on their bodies and minds.

Acupuncture and Digestive Disorders:

The efficacy of acupuncture in treating digestive diseases is becoming more widely acknowledged; it provides an alternative to traditional medical therapies.

The technique includes improving blood flow, controlling the gastrointestinal system, and stimulating particular sites related to the digestive organs. Acupuncture is a potential treatment for those with irritable bowel syndrome (IBS), acid reflux, and chronic constipation.

Acupuncture seeks to improve digestive function, relieve symptoms, and improve overall gastrointestinal health by re-establishing the body's energy flow equilibrium.

Using Acupuncture to Promote Fertility: A Whole Approach

Acupuncture has become known as a comprehensive and integrated method to improve reproductive health for couples who are having trouble conceiving.

Reducing stress, enhancing blood flow to the reproductive organs, and regulating hormone imbalances are all goals of the therapy, as they can all affect fertility. To maximize the odds of success, acupuncture is frequently combined with assisted reproductive technologies, such as in vitro fertilization (IVF).

According to research, couples receiving fertility treatments may experience higher pregnancy and live birth rates after receiving acupuncture. Furthermore, acupuncture offers a holistic method of assisting individuals and couples in their conception process by addressing the mental and physical components of fertility.

These acupuncture applications highlight the treatment's adaptability and profound effects on a range of health and well-being issues. As complementary therapy, acupuncture is becoming more and more well-known for its capacity to treat a variety of ailments and provide people with a customized, all-encompassing approach to recovery and good health.

CHAPTER 6

CONDITIONS TREATED WITH REFLEXOLOGY
Reflexology for Relaxation and Stress Reduction:

Reflexology is a holistic therapy that uses pressure on certain areas of the hands, feet, or ears to encourage relaxation and lessen stress. This age-old method derives from the idea that these regions represent various bodily systems and organs.

Applying pressure is believed to encourage balance and encourage the flow of energy.

Reflexology relieves tension and promotes deep relaxation in the context of relaxation and stress reduction. The nervous system is activated by focusing on particular reflex spots, which lowers the release of stress chemicals. Because reflexology is a mild and non-invasive method, it is well-liked by those looking for all-natural solutions to reduce stress and enhance their general well-being.

Enhancing Your Reflexology and Sleep:

In today's fast-paced society, many people suffer from sleep disorders and disturbances. An alternative to pharmaceuticals for enhancing the quality of sleep is reflexology.

It is thought that stimulating specific reflex sites might soothe the nervous system and improve sleep patterns. Reflexology seeks to balance the body's energy and foster calm by concentrating on particular regions linked to relaxation, such as the solar plexus and pituitary gland reflex sites. Reflexology is a supplemental treatment for people with sleep-related problems since it can help with sleep duration, insomnia, and general quality of sleep when done regularly.

Handling Prolonged Pain via Reflexology:

Reflexology is becoming more widely accepted as an adjunctive treatment for illnesses including chronic pain. The method works on the tenet that particular reflex sites correlate to various bodily sections, including pain-affected locations. Reflexology works by applying pressure to these reflex sites to reduce pain and enhance well-being.

Reflexology can be used to target problematic areas and encourage the body's natural healing processes in cases of chronic pain, such as arthritis or back pain. Furthermore, reflexology's capacity to promote relaxation can aid in the management of pain by easing tense muscles and enhancing blood flow. Reflexology can be a useful part of an all-encompassing pain management regimen, but it is not a replacement for medical care.

Using Reflexology to Improve Circulation:

Since circulation keeps waste products out of the body and guarantees that nutrients and oxygen reach the cells, it is essential to overall health. By focusing on particular reflex sites connected to the cardiovascular system, reflexology is thought to improve circulation.

Reflexology manipulates and applies pressure to these spots to enhance blood flow and support vascular health. Better oxygenation of tissues, higher energy levels, and enhanced cardiovascular function are just a few advantages of improved circulation. Reflexology is a highly sought-after therapy for individuals seeking to boost their circulatory system and promote optimal health due to its holistic approach to well-being. Frequent sessions could support the preservation of a harmonious and balanced energy flow throughout the body.

CHAPTER 7

INCLUDING REFLEXOLOGY AND ACUPUNCTURE IN WELLNESS PRACTICES
The Functions of Acupuncture and Reflexology in Holistic Health:

In the pursuit of optimum well-being, holistic health takes into account the full person—body, mind, spirit, and emotions. Reflexology and acupuncture are essential parts of holistic health techniques, providing different viewpoints on healing.

With its roots in traditional Chinese medicine, acupuncture stimulates energy flow and restores balance by inserting tiny needles into certain body locations. Conversely, reflexology emphasizes applying pressure to particular locations on the hands, feet, or ears to facilitate healing in the corresponding bodily parts.

The underlying idea behind these techniques is that emotional or physical imbalances can result from interruptions in the body's natural energy pathways.

Reflexology and acupuncture both aim to bring the body back into balance by treating the underlying causes of illnesses as well as their symptoms. These therapies provide a holistic view of health and wellness by acknowledging the interdependence of different body systems.

Including Traditional Chinese Medicine in Everyday Activities:

A comprehensive framework for comprehending health and illness is provided by Traditional Chinese Medicine (TCM), which includes reflexology and acupuncture as essential techniques.

According to TCM, the body is a dynamic system in which energy channels, or meridians, carry the life force, or Qi.

The goal of acupuncture is to restore harmony by balancing the flow of Qi and preventing or treating illnesses. Though different from TCM, reflexology addresses energy imbalances by stimulating certain reflex spots, which is a comparable approach.

Adopting habits that promote general well-being is a necessary part of incorporating TCM into daily life. This could involve adopting a diet based on Chinese nutritional principles, using herbal medicines, and engaging in Qigong or Tai Chi exercises to improve Qi flow. By accepting these components, people can actively practice self-care, encouraging equilibrium and averting imbalances that could result in disease.

Mind-Body Link: Using Breathwork and Meditation in Addition to Acupuncture and Reflexology

A key component of holistic health is the mind-body connection, and techniques like breathwork and meditation work well in conjunction with reflexology and acupuncture. Through the practice of mindfulness, meditation raises awareness of one's thoughts, feelings, and physical sensations. Meditation strengthens the healing effects of acupuncture or reflexology sessions by promoting a calm state of mind and strengthening the mind-body connection.

Another effective technique is breathwork, which uses deliberate control over breathing patterns to affect both mental and physical conditions. Intentional breathing enhances the relaxation response and aids in the release of tension and stress when used in conjunction with reflexology or acupuncture. Because they target both the mental and physical components of well-being, these activities are complementary to one another.

In a nutshell the integration of reflexology and acupuncture within holistic medical practices offers a variety of approaches to overall wellness. People can embark on a profound and life-changing path toward optimal well-being by realizing the holistic nature of health, embracing the mind-body link through breathwork and meditation, and applying traditional Chinese medicine concepts to daily life.

CHAPTER 8

SELECTING A PRACTITIONER AND SAFETY ISSUES
Locating an Accredited Acupuncturist:

To guarantee a secure and efficient acupuncture treatment, it is essential to locate a skilled practitioner. Begin by investigating local practitioners who hold licenses and certifications from the appropriate regulatory agencies.

These groups frequently establish guidelines for moral behavior, instruction, and training. An experienced acupuncturist usually has a degree in acupuncture or traditional Chinese medicine and has received a lot of training. Think about asking friends or medical professionals who have had good experiences with acupuncture for advice. Furthermore, internet reviews and testimonials can provide information about a practitioner's track record and degree of effectiveness in treating certain ailments.

Choosing an Expert Reflexologist:

For best effects, a qualified practitioner is needed for reflexology, a therapeutic technique that includes applying pressure to particular points on the hands, feet, or ears. Seek out reflexologists who are accredited by respectable reflexology societies and who have undergone professional training. Techniques in anatomy, physiology, and reflexology are frequently covered in training programs.

Think about choosing medical professionals who specialize in treating ailments or health issues that are pertinent to your needs. You can choose a reflexologist with a track record of providing safe and successful treatments by using online reviews, personal recommendations, and referrals from medical professionals.

Safety Measures and Possible Hazards:

Although skilled practitioners can safely practice acupuncture and reflexology, it's important to be aware of potential hazards and safety precautions. To lower the risk of infection, make sure your acupuncturist uses sterile, disposable needles. Give your doctor a thorough medical history that includes all current prescriptions, allergies, and medical concerns. Expectant clients need to let their acupuncturist know that some acupuncture sites might not be safe to use while pregnant. Although reflexology is typically safe, anyone with specific foot disorders, like infections or open wounds, should use caution.

Both reflexology and acupuncture may cause modest adverse effects, such as bruises, pain, or a brief exacerbation of symptoms. However, when therapies are given by trained doctors, major side effects are uncommon. Inform your practitioner as soon as possible if you have any unexpected discomfort or negative interactions. Maintaining regular contact with your healthcare practitioner is also crucial, particularly if you are receiving reflexology or acupuncture in addition to traditional medical treatments. Prioritize your safety and well-being at all times by selecting trustworthy professionals and adhering to their advice throughout treatment.

CHAPTER 9

CASE STUDIES AND SUCCESS STORIES IN
Actual Reflexology and Acupuncture Experiences:

Within complementary and alternative medicine, acupuncture and reflexology have attracted a lot of interest due to their ability to treat a wide range of physical and psychological conditions. Experiences with these techniques in real life frequently demonstrate the significant positive effects they can have on people's well-being. Consider the case of Sarah, a lady who endured years of suffering from persistent headaches. Her condition improved temporarily with traditional treatments, but she found a long-term answer with acupuncture sessions. Sarah's story highlights how individualized and comprehensive acupuncture is since practitioners frequently customize treatments to target particular health issues.

In a similar vein, reflexology has been mentioned in the accounts of numerous people who have used it to find relief from ailments like chronic pain, stress, and worry. John, a corporate worker, used reflexology as a coping mechanism for the stress that came with his hard work. Regular sessions brought him not only physical relaxation but also advantages in his general state of mind. These actual interactions demonstrate how adaptable reflexology is in fostering emotional and physical balance.

Case Studies Illustrating the Success of Treatment:

Examining individual situations helps to clarify the efficacy of reflexology and acupuncture. Take Emily's example, a middle-aged woman who struggles with worry and sleeplessness. After experiencing minimal success with conventional medical techniques, she decided to investigate acupuncture. Emily's symptoms significantly decreased in frequency and intensity throughout several treatments. This case study demonstrates how acupuncture can provide alleviation for diseases that are frequently associated with imbalances by correcting the body's energy flow.

Likewise, reflexology has proven to be effective in managing chronic pain. Mark, who has had lower back pain for a long time, looked into reflexology as an additional treatment option. He felt relaxation and greater movement through specific foot reflex sites. These case studies demonstrate how these approaches can supplement traditional medical treatments in addition to highlighting their therapeutic potential.

Patient Testimonials and Life-Changing Experiences:

Testimonials from patients are potent storytelling devices that shed light on the life-changing experiences people have with reflexology and acupuncture. For example, Maria had been suffering from stomach problems for years before she started acupuncture. Her testimonies underscore the beneficial effects on her bodily well-being as well as the psychological and emotional transformations that came with the healing process. These testimonies highlight the holistic aspect of these activities and recognize that they can treat several aspects of well-being.

In a similar vein, people relate their experiences with reflexology, highlighting the wider influence on their lives. Reflexology sessions provided James, a busy executive, with comfort and greater focus, which eventually improved their work-life balance. When taken as a whole, these testimonies depict acupuncture and reflexology as more than just remedies for certain conditions; rather, they act as catalysts for complete changes that promote a feeling of health that goes beyond the clinic.

CHAPTER 10

ACUPUNCTURE AND REFLEXOLOGY'S FUTURE
Investigating Higher Consciousness Levels:

Higher states of consciousness are frequently explored in advanced chakra techniques. Those who work with their chakras more deeply may become more aware of their surroundings and have wider perspectives.

Deep meditation states, spiritual epiphanies, and a strong bond with the universal energy could all be examples of this. Techniques like visualization, breathwork, and meditation are used to raise consciousness and let in transcendent experiences. People who study advanced chakras frequently report feeling more attuned to the cosmos, having better intuition, and having a profound awareness of their spiritual being.

Chakras and the Awakening of Kundalini:

An essential component of advanced chakra practices is kundalini awakening. It is thought that kundalini is a latent energy that lies at the base of the spine and may be led through the energy centers and awakened through a variety of chakra activities.

This awakening is sometimes compared to a strong energy rush that causes deep awareness transformation and enhanced spiritual experiences.

The complex relationship between Kundalini energy and the chakras is responsible for each chakra's role in the overall process of spiritual development. Working with this powerful energy, advanced practitioners strive for a harmonic ascent in line with the chakras' opening and balance.

Chakra Activation Using Mantras and Sound:

Mantras and sound are effective tools for activating chakras in advanced chakra activities. Every chakra has a unique set of vibrations and sounds, and practitioners employ particular mantras or sounds to connect with and open these energy centers. Chanting, tuning forks, or singing bowls are some examples of instruments that can be used for this. You can also listen to particular frequencies.

It is thought that the resonance of these sounds produces balances and opens the chakras, allowing energy to freely circulate throughout the body. Chakra's work gains a dynamic and vibrational dimension from this acoustic technique, making it a more multisensory and comprehensive practice.

Retreats and Workshops on Chakra Healing:

Retreats and seminars on chakra healing provide immersive opportunities for people who want to learn more about and practice advanced chakra work. These gatherings offer a nurturing setting where attendees can pick up knowledge from seasoned instructors, partake in supervised exercises, and exchange perspectives with like-minded people.

A range of activities, including energy healing techniques, meditation sessions, and in-depth talks on complex chakra principles, may be included in workshops. Retreats, which are frequently held in tranquil, natural settings, combine spiritual teachings with the restorative power of nature to give a holistic approach to chakra healing.

Customized Chakra Tours & Ongoing Development:

More advanced chakra activities place a strong emphasis on individual growth paths and ongoing development. Since every person's chakra system is different, practitioners customize their techniques to target certain imbalances or areas of personal growth.

This could entail concentrating on specific chakras, blending different methods, and modifying the practice over time. The journey transforms into a dynamic process of ongoing self-improvement and self-discovery, inspiring people to advance spiritually and incorporate chakra work into their everyday lives.

To successfully negotiate the intricacies of advanced chakra practices and guarantee a well-rounded and long-lasting approach to personal development, individuals frequently seek out individualized instruction from knowledgeable mentors or spiritual instructors.

These elements work together to provide a thorough grasp of advanced chakra activities, emphasizing the breadth and depth of the spiritual journey people experience while delving into the subtleties of their energy centers.

THE END

Made in the USA
Columbia, SC
25 July 2024

39309519R00033